UNCAGING
THE MIND

SHANI T. NIGHT

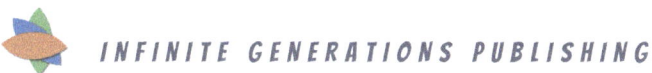

INFINITE GENERATIONS PUBLISHING

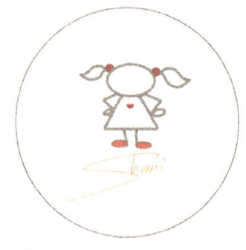

Paperback ISBN: 978-1-953364-74-6

Infinite Generations
137 National Plaza, STE 300
National Harbor, MD 20745

Printed in the United States of America

Art by Canva
Cover Design by: I Howard and D. Spruill

POSITIVE MEDIA, HAPPY LIFE

WWW.INFINITEGENERATIONS.COM

From the Author

Written to help you move from simply surviving... to soulfully living.

This book offers the why, the how, and the hope from someone who's done the inner work, walked through the fire, and found the light. Now, I'm handing that light back to you.

May these pages remind you that your freedom was never lost—only waiting to be reclaimed.

With love,
Shani T. Night
Certified Happiness Coach & Joy Advocate

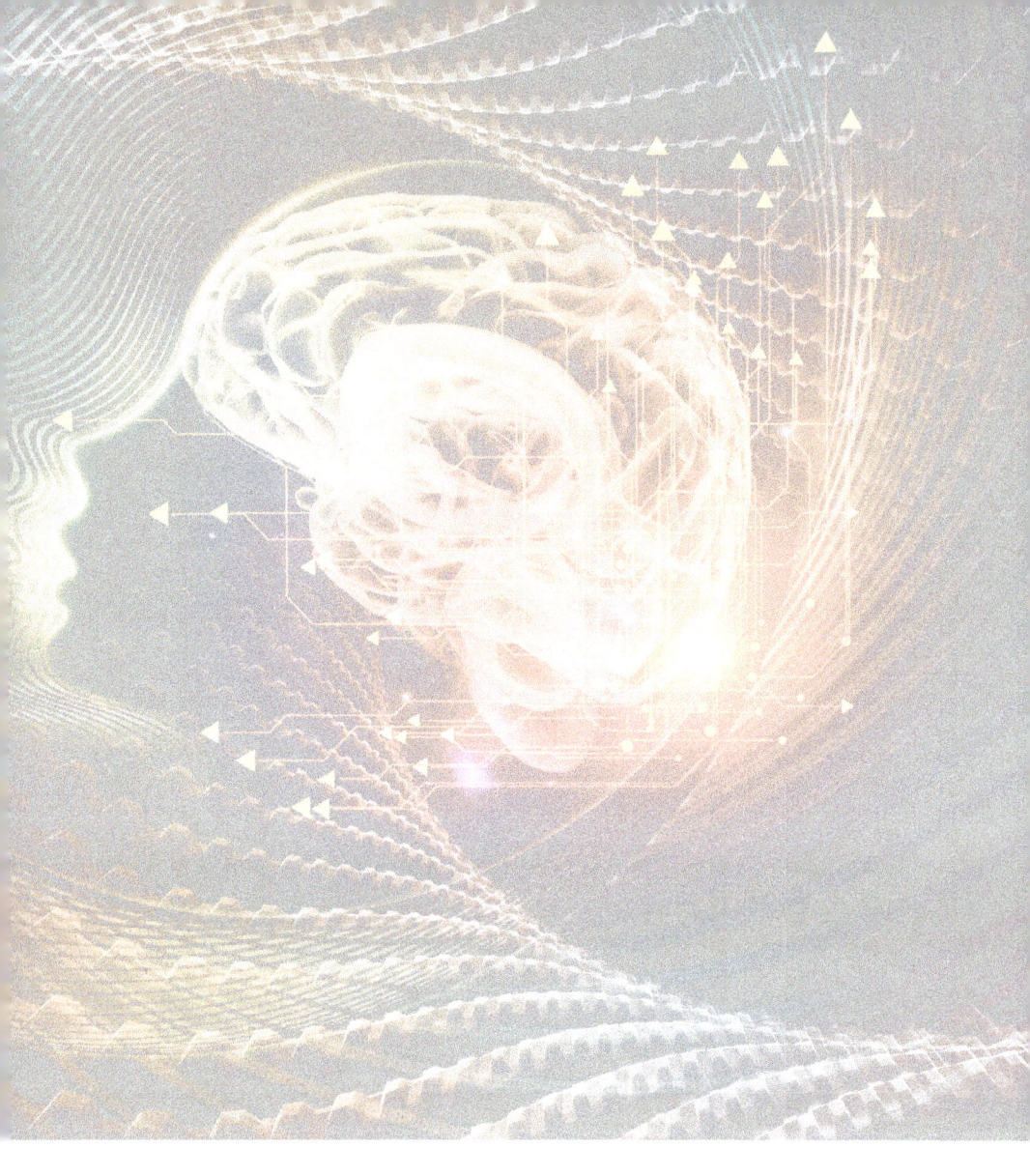

"The mind—what a tricky place when left untended. It feeds on the unseen, the unspoken, and often replays what feels broken. Yet it remains a powerful muscle of memory—one that can imprison or free, depending on how we care for it."

SHANI T. NIGHT

Dear Reader:

Thank you for your purchase.
I hope you enjoy Uncaging the Mind: From Survival to Soulful Living.

Please share a review of this book on Amazon.

Visit my website for more content, discounts, contests, giveaways,
and/or a free consult.
www.shanitnight.com

Follow Shani Night:
instagram.com/shaninight
www.facebook.com/ShaniTNight
I post daily/weekly positive messages.

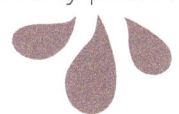

"Be soft with yourself.
You're still blooming."

SHANI T. NIGHT

Special Dedication

To my Aunt Dot,
who gave me permission to be
before the world knew how to say it out loud.

At a time when I was quietly folding myself into who others
needed me to be, you handed me the courage to ask my own
heart for direction. You didn't just encourage authenticity—you
demanded it, long before it became a buzzword.

Your words cracked open the first door to freedom:
"Be unapologetically you."
I've been walking through that door ever since.

This book lives because of that moment.
Thank you, Aunt Dot, for helping me uncage my mind.

"I aspire to be the best part of me."
SHANI T. NIGHT

🌿 Dedication

For anyone who has ever felt the grip of fear, the ache of self-doubt, or the heavy weight of expectations.

To those who've known the quiet ache of being caged, unseen, or unheard—
This book is for you.

May it guide you back to your power, your light, and your freedom.
May you remember who you were before the world told you otherwise.
May you rise, soften, and soar in your truth.

This is your power.
This is your light.
This is for your return to joy.
This is for your soul.
This is for your freedom.

With love,
Shani T. Night

Healing is not a linear process.
SHANI T. NIGHT

TABLE OF CONTENTS

"The road less traveled can lead to marvelous things."

SHANI T. NIGHT

INTRODUCTION: THE INVISIBLE CAGE

INTRODUCTION: THE INVISIBLE CAGE

I didn't always know I was caged. Not at first.

It started somewhere around my teenage years, maybe high school, when the feeling of *not being enough* settled quietly into my spirit like a fog. It wasn't loud or dramatic. It was subtle, made up of small moments that chipped away at my joy, my peace, and my confidence.

I can still remember the younger version of me before the cage formed. She was bold, imaginative, and sure of her worth.
She believed she could be anything. That inner child still lives inside me—her light dimmed for a while, but never fully went out.

Somewhere along the way, I started believing other people's opinions of me more than my own truth. The weight of expectations, comparisons, and silent judgment wrapped around me like invisible bars. And maybe I stepped into the cage willingly, out of self-doubt or a need to belong, but I definitely stopped living as *me*.

I became who I thought I was supposed to be. I began reacting to the expectations of others, not just meeting them, but often exceeding them, even when they dimmed my light.

I followed instead of led, shrinking parts of myself to fit molds I was never meant to occupy.

INTRODUCTION: THE INVISIBLE CAGE

I became who I thought I was supposed to be.

Piece by piece, I shaped myself around the expectations of others—teachers, society, seasonal friends, and even those called true friends.

I didn't realize it at the time, but I had stopped asking, Who am I really? Instead, I started reacting, responding to the needs, desires, and silent rules placed upon me. I didn't just meet expectations; I surpassed them, thinking that was the key to love, acceptance, and belonging.

But in doing so, I began to lose pieces of myself. I followed instead of led. I blended in when I was meant to stand out.
I quieted my voice to keep the peace. And somewhere along the way, I began shrinking, not just in action, but in spirit.

I didn't realize that the praise I received wasn't affirming my truth; it was affirming a version of me that wasn't whole. A version that was performing, pleasing, and perfecting, but not truly living.

This book, and the journey I share within it, is about returning to the you that existed before the world told you who to be. It's about uncaging your mind, reclaiming your joy, and learning to lead from within.

Uncaging began when I made the brave decision to walk away from the noise, from the people, environments, and mental patterns that no longer served my becoming. I started asking myself:
Who am I without the fear? Without the guilt? Without the pressure?

The subconscious is the quiet witness you never knew you had—watching as you drift further from your truth. Even when you aren't fully aware, it remembers who you are and gently tries to guide you back home.

SHANI T. NIGHT

INTRODUCTION: THE INVISIBLE CAGE

It wasn't a perfect process. There were missteps and painful lessons, mistakes that taught me more than any success ever could. But even in the mess, I could feel something beautiful taking shape. Like a diamond in the rough, I was forming under pressure, gaining clarity and strength with each turn inward.

Now, I live differently.

I am fully, unapologetically *me*.
I protect my peace.
I honor my time.
I live with deep intention and radical self-acceptance.

The truth is, life will always bring new challenges. Just when you think you've figured it all out, another layer of growth unfolds. But I no longer see that as a setback. I see it as a sign that I'm alive and evolving—and exactly where I need to be.

This book is not a perfect map. It's not a set of rules. It's a reflection of how I *uncaged my mind* and returned to myself. It's honest, open, and filled with the same hope I offer my clients and my own soul every day.

So read with an open heart.
Take what speaks to you.
Leave what doesn't.

And most of all, remember:
The light inside you has never gone out. It may be dimmed, buried, or quiet, but it's still there.

Let this be your invitation to rise. To come home to yourself.
To uncage your mind—and finally, live free.

AWARENESS

Awareness is the conscious knowledge, recognition, and understanding of something, whether it's a thought, feeling, behavior, environment, or experience. It's the ability to notice what's happening both inside of you and around you without judgment.

From a happiness coach's perspective, awareness is the first step to transformation.

It's what allows you to:
- Recognize limiting beliefs or thought patterns
- Tune in to your emotions and needs
- Make intentional choices instead of reactive ones
- Pause before you speak or act
- Create space for growth, healing, and clarity

When you're aware, you become the observer of your life—not just a participant. And in that space of observation, you can begin to shift what no longer serves you and lean into what does.

YOU CAN'T RECEIVE WHAT YOU'RE NOT OPEN TO

A package can be delivered to your doorstep... but if the door stays closed, it remains untouched.

A phone call can come through...but if you don't answer, you miss the connection.

Life works the same way.

Love, healing, guidance, new beginnings—they don't force their way in.
They knock.
They call.
They wait for your openness.

✨ An open mind allows you to see what you couldn't before.
✨ An open heart allows you to feel what you've been afraid to receive.

So today, ask yourself:

Am I truly open to what I say I want?
Or am I standing at the door, locked by fear, pride, or old stories?

You don't have to be perfect. You just have to be willing.
Leave the door cracked.
Answer the call.
Something beautiful might be waiting.

"*Awareness is the quiet voice within that says, 'This is not who you are.' It doesn't shout or shame, it simply reminds you to return to your truth, and rise with grace.*"

SHANI T. NIGHT

CHAPTER 1:
RECOGNIZE THE CAGE

RECOGNIZE THE CAGE

You can't break free from something you don't know you're trapped in.

One of the greatest acts of self-love is acknowledging the invisible bars that have quietly shaped your choices, your voice, and your sense of worth. These cages aren't built overnight—they're crafted over time by fear, by judgment, by inherited beliefs, and by a world that often tells us who we should be instead of helping us discover who we truly are.

I often tell my clients: *"You're not broken—you're just caged."* And the first step to freedom is recognizing the walls around you.

The Subtle Shape of a Cage

Cages don't always look like suffering. Sometimes they look like success with burnout, smiles with no peace, or a perfect life that doesn't feel like your own. They can be hard to recognize because they're often made of thoughts that feel true:

- "I have to make everyone happy."
- "If I slow down, I'll fall behind."
- "I'm not good enough to go after what I really want."
- "This is just how life is."

But let me ask you this:
Who told you that? And when did you start believing it?

We carry mental programming passed down from parents, teachers, religion, culture, and even trauma. Over time, these programs become our "truths," and we unconsciously build our lives around them.

These beliefs shape what we think we're capable of. They convince us that being free is unsafe, that being happy is selfish, or that we don't deserve more than what we have.

That's the cage.

RECOGNIZE THE CAGE

Identifying Your Cage

So how do you know if you're caged?

Ask yourself:
- Am I living in alignment with what truly brings me joy?
- Do I feel stuck in patterns I don't understand?
- Do I silence myself to keep the peace?
- Do I feel like I'm constantly performing for approval?

Your answers will reveal the shape of your particular cage.

Some cages are built from:

- **Self-doubt:** A relentless whisper telling you you're not enough.
- **Guilt:** The belief that your joy must come at the cost of someone else's comfort.
- **Comparison:** Measuring your worth against someone else's highlight reel.
- **People-pleasing:** Basing your decisions on how others might react.
- **Fear of failure:** Believing that trying and failing is worse than not trying at all.
- **Perfectionism:** Thinking you have to "get it all right" before you can be worthy of peace.

You don't need to have all of these to feel caged. Just one is enough to limit your freedom.

RECOGNIZE THE CAGE

Naming the Cage Weakens It

What we cannot name, we cannot change. But once you name it —once you say, "This is fear" or "This is shame" or "This is a belief I inherited, not one I chose", you begin to loosen its grip.

It's like turning on the light in a dark room. The monsters shrink.

One of my clients, a brilliant woman in her 40s, spent years overworking to prove herself. She told me, "If I stop, I'll disappear." When we peeled back the layers, we found an old childhood memory of being ignored unless she was accomplishing something. Her cage was built from the belief that *being* wasn't enough—only *doing* made her lovable.

When she recognized that cage, everything started to shift. She didn't need to tear down her life to be free. She just had to start choosing differently—from awareness, not autopilot.

The Courage to See

It takes courage to look at your life honestly. It's easier to stay busy. It's easier to distract, numb, or blame.

But you are not here for a half-life. You are here to be fully alive, fully expressed, and fully *you*.

Recognizing your cage is not an act of weakness, it's the beginning of power.

Because once you see it, you can question it.
Once you question it, you can challenge it.
And once you challenge it, you can change it.

RECOGNIZE THE CAGE

A Gentle Invitation

As you finish this chapter, I invite you to pause and reflect, not to judge yourself, but to become lovingly aware.

Ask yourself:
- What thoughts, beliefs, or fears keep showing up in my life like old songs on repeat?
- What would I do or say differently if I truly felt free?
- What part of me longs to come alive?

This is not about fixing yourself. You are not broken.
This is about freeing yourself, because the cage was never your home.
Your spirit was meant to soar.

"Have enough courage to heal."
SHANI T. NIGHT

"Healing begins when you face the clouds, not flee from them."

SHANI T. NIGHT

REFLECTION EXERCISE:

- Write down five "I should..." statements that often run through your mind.
- Next to each one, ask: Who told me this? and Is it true?
- Rewrite each statement into an empowering truth.

Example:

- "I should always say yes to be liked." → "I can say no with love and still be worthy."

"*Awareness is the light that shines on your truth—it doesn't change the path, but it helps you walk it with your eyes open.*"

SHANI T. NIGHT

CHAPTER 2:
CHALLENGE THE NARRATIVE

CHALLENGE THE NARRATIVE

Once you recognize the cage, the next step is realizing something even more powerful:

You are not the story you've been telling yourself.

The stories we carry—about who we are, what we're capable of, and what's possible for us—are like invisible scripts. We read from them without question, often unaware that they were written by someone else or shaped by moments that no longer define us.

But here's the truth:

You can edit the script. You can write a new story.
And it all starts with challenging the old one.

The Voice in Your Head

Everyone has an inner narrator. Sometimes, it sounds like a helpful guide. Other times, it sounds like a harsh critic or a fearful child.

- *"I always mess things up."*
- *"They'll leave me if I don't keep them happy."*
- *"I'm too old, too late, too far behind."*
- *"People like me don't get to have that kind of life."*

These aren't facts.
They're beliefs—usually absorbed, not chosen.

They were often born in moments of pain, shame, rejection, or fear. Maybe someone criticized you harshly as a child. Maybe you failed once and were made to feel like it defined you. Maybe the world around you reflected back a narrow view of what success, beauty, or worth looked like.

And so, your mind did what minds do:
It created a narrative to protect you from future pain.
But protection isn't the same as truth.

CHALLENGE THE NARRATIVE

The Stories We Tell

Let me introduce you to a powerful happiness tool I teach my clients:

The Thought-Truth Shift.
Step 1: Name the story.
Step 2: Ask, *Is this absolutely true?*
Step 3: Shift the story to something more empowering.

Let's take an example:

- **Thought:** "I'm not creative. I've never been artistic."
- **Truth Check:** Is this really true? Have I *never* been creative? Or is this a belief formed by comparison or criticism?
- **Shifted Narrative:** "I express creativity in my own way. I don't need to be Picasso to be creative."

Another:
- Thought: "I'm too much. I need to tone myself down."
- Truth Check: Who said you're too much? Or were they just uncomfortable with your light?
- Shifted Narrative: "My fullness is a gift. I don't have to shrink to fit small spaces."

"The mind—what a tricky place when left untended. It feeds on the unseen, the unspoken, and often replays what feels broken. Yet it remains a powerful muscle of memory—one that can imprison or free, depending on how we care for it."

CHALLENGE THE NARRATIVE

Challenging the Voice of Fear

Many of the stories we carry are rooted in fear, fear of rejection, of failure, of not being enough. But here's something liberating:

Fear often masquerades as truth, but it's just a protective voice trying to keep you from discomfort.
We have to learn to *witness* that voice, not obey it.

- Instead of, "*I'll never be successful,*" ask, "What does success look like for me—and who told me I couldn't have it?"
- Instead of, "*I'm not as good as them,*" ask, "What if I'm just different, not lesser?"
- Instead of, "*I can't change,*" ask, "What small step can I take today to prove that wrong?"

When you begin to question fear-based thoughts, you invite in the possibility of freedom.

✦ Small shifts can lead to soul-stirring deep transformation. Choose with intention. ✦
SHANI T. NIGHT

CHALLENGE THE NARRATIVE

The Brain's Comfort with Familiar Stories

The brain loves what's familiar. even if it's painful. So don't be surprised if old stories cling to you like second skin. They've been with you for years. But just because they've stayed doesn't mean they get to lead.

Freedom begins when you decide:
Just because I've believed it for a long time doesn't mean I have to believe it today.

Rewrite, Reclaim, Reignite

Here's the beautiful part: Once you challenge the old narrative, you make space for a new one.
And this time, you get to choose the words.

You are not too late.
You are not too broken.
You are not too loud, too quiet, too much, or not enough.
You are **becoming**—and that is more powerful than being perfect.

A Happiness Coach's Reminder

I've worked with people from every walk of life—CEOs, single parents, artists, teachers, students—and what I've seen is universal:
Every single person has a story they've been living that's smaller than their truth.

The work of uncaging the mind is not about bulldozing your past. It's about lovingly turning toward the stories that shaped you and *saying, Thank you for trying to protect me. But I don't need you anymore.*

"The mind, like the body, is brilliantly designed to protect us. And in the moment, that protection can be life-saving. But when the moment has passed and the mind stays in defense mode—unable to adapt because it was never given the tools—that same protection can become a cage. Healing begins when we gently teach the mind that it is safe to grow, to soften, and to begin again."

SHANI T. NIGHT

REFLECTION EXERCISE: REWRITING YOUR NARRATIVE

1. Write down a limiting belief you often think.
Example: "I'm not smart enough to start a business."
2. Ask yourself: Is this 100% true? Where did it come from?
Who planted that seed?
3. Rewrite the story.
 Example: "I'm capable of learning what I need to know. Many successful people started with no experience—I'm allowed to start too."
4. Say it aloud.
 Words have power. Let your ears hear the new truth.

_____

_____

_____

_____

_____

_____

_____

_____

_____

_____

_____

_____

_____

_____

You don't need anyone's permission to change the story. You are the author now. And the next chapter? It's one of love, liberation, and truth.

ACCEPTANCE

Acceptance is the act of embracing reality as it is—without resistance, denial, or judgment. It means acknowledging your thoughts, feelings, experiences, and circumstances without trying to fight them or force them to be something they're not.

From a happiness coach's perspective, **acceptance is not giving up, it's choosing peace over struggle.** It's the moment you stop arguing with life and start living it fully, even when it doesn't look exactly the way you imagined.

Acceptance allows you to:
- Make peace with the past
- Release the need for control
- Show yourself compassion
- Break free from shame, guilt, or resentment
- Open the door to healing and transformation

When you accept something, you're not saying it's ideal or permanent—you're simply saying: **"This is what is, and I choose to respond with clarity, grace, and purpose."**

✦ *Acceptance is not weakness—it's wisdom wrapped in softness. It's the soil in which peace, growth, and happiness take root.* ✦

CHAPTER 3:
CULTIVATE SELF-COMPASSION

CULTIVATE SELF-COMPASSION

If challenging the narrative is about changing the story, then cultivating self-compassion is about changing the *tone*. It's not enough to replace negative beliefs, we have to learn to speak to ourselves with the same tenderness we offer others.

Because if the voice in your head still sounds like a bully, even your most empowering thoughts will feel like pressure instead of peace.

Self-compassion is the key that unlocks lasting freedom.

The Inner Critic vs. The Inner Caregiver

We all have an inner critic. You know the voice:
- *"Why did you do that? That was so dumb."*
- *"You're always messing things up."*
- *"You should be further along by now."*

That voice may sound familiar because it often echoes what we heard growing up—whether from teachers, friends, society, or even ourselves in our most vulnerable moments.

But here's the truth:
You can't shame yourself into healing.
You can't criticize yourself into growth.
And you definitely can't hate yourself into happiness.

You need a new voice. A gentler one.

A wise inner caregiver who says things like:
- *"It's okay. You're learning."*
- *"You tried your best today, and that's enough."*
- *"You're not broken. You're becoming."*

CULTIVATE SELF-COMPASSION

The Cost of Self-Criticism

As a happiness coach, I often ask my clients:
Would you talk to a child the way you talk to yourself?

Usually, their eyes well up. Because deep down, they know they've been carrying around unrealistic expectations, punishing self-talk, and perfectionism disguised as motivation. But self-criticism doesn't push us forward, it paralyzes us. It fuels anxiety, low self-worth, burnout, and even depression. It keeps us in the cage.

Self-compassion is the antidote.

What Self-Compassion Isn't

Let's clear up a common misconception: **Self-compassion is not self-pity. It's not laziness. It's not letting yourself off the hook.**

It's about giving yourself permission to be human.
You can acknowledge mistakes while still loving yourself.
You can strive for more while honoring where you are.
You can be a work in progress and still be worthy of joy.

Self-compassion is fierce. It says:
- "I'm doing the best I can with what I have."
- "I won't abandon myself, even when I'm hurting."
- "My value isn't up for debate."

CULTIVATE SELF-COMPASSION

The Three Pillars of Self-Compassion
(adapted from the work of Dr. Kristin Neff)

- Mindfulness - Be present with your pain instead of ignoring it or blowing it out of proportion.

- Common Humanity - Remind yourself: I'm not alone. Everyone struggles. Being imperfect is part of being human.

- Self-Kindness - Speak to yourself like you would to someone you love. Use kind, encouraging, and forgiving language.

Compassion as a Daily Practice

Self-compassion isn't something you "achieve." It's a muscle you build. A practice you return to. A way of being that transforms how you experience life.

Here are a few practices to get you started:

- **Place your hand on your heart** when you're upset. Say, "This is hard. And I'm here for myself."

- **Write a letter to yourself** from the perspective of someone who loves you unconditionally.

- **Notice when you're slipping into comparison** or guilt. Pause and ask, "What do I need right now?"

- **Forgive yourself often**—for not knowing, for not doing it perfectly, for simply being human.

CULTIVATE SELF-COMPASSION

A Happiness Coach's Insight

I've watched clients transform—not because they reached their goals faster, but because they learned to love themselves *while* reaching for them.

They stopped waiting until they were "better," "thinner," "more successful," or "perfect."
And they started celebrating the brave, messy, beautiful humans they already were.

Freedom doesn't come from becoming someone else. It comes from embracing who you are with kindness.

"You cannot heal what you refuse to hold.
The sky clears not by force, but by facing
the clouds with an open heart."

SHANI T. NIGHT

REFLECTION EXERCISE: YOUR COMPASSIONATE VOICE

1. Think of a recent moment when you were hard on yourself.
Maybe you missed a deadline, said something you regretted, or felt "off."

2. Now imagine your best friend came to you with that same problem.
What would you say to them?

3. **Write those exact words to yourself.**
Yes, you deserve that same grace.

4. Post it somewhere you'll see it often.
Compassion is not a luxury. It's your lifeline.

_____

_____

_____

_____

_____

_____

_____

_____

_____

_____

_____

_____

_____

_____

_____

Self-compassion isn't a soft skill, it's soul fuel.
When you speak to yourself with gentleness, you give your inner light permission to shine again. And slowly, day by day, the cage begins to open.

Next, we'll explore what it means to <u>Choose Presence Over Perfection,</u> and how doing so can finally set you free from the myth of "getting it all right."

"Go gently inward, not to fix, but to listen. The answers you seek are already whispering beneath the noise."

SHANI T. NIGHT

CHAPTER 4:
CHOOSE PRESENCE OVER PERFECTION

CHOOSE PRESENCE OVER PERFECTION

Perfection is the prettiest cage of all. It's polished. It's praised. It looks like something worth pursuing. But make no mistake—**it's still a trap.**

Perfectionism convinces us that we'll be happy *when*:
- We lose the weight.
- We land the job.
- We fix the relationship.
- We have it "all together."

But what's the cost?

A life spent chasing an illusion, while the present quietly slips through our fingers.

The Perfection Illusion

Let's be honest, perfection is a moving target. No matter how much you achieve, there's always more to fix, improve, or become. And while you're busy striving for flawless, you're missing *life*.

Here's the truth:

Perfection isn't real. But presence is.
And presence is where joy lives.

CHOOSE PRESENCE OVER PERFECTION

Why We Chase It Anyway

Perfectionism is often rooted in fear:
- Fear of judgment
- Fear of failure
- Fear of not being enough

It can even be a trauma response—trying to control what's around us because something inside us feels unsafe or unworthy. We think if we just get everything "right," maybe we'll finally earn love, acceptance, or peace. But peace doesn't come from control. It comes from surrender. **From being, not doing.**

The Gift of Presence

Presence is not passive.
It's powerful.

It means slowing down enough to feel the moment. To hear the laughter, taste the coffee, notice the sunlight on your skin.

It means showing up for your life with your *whole self*, not just the curated version you think is worthy.

When we are present:
- We release the pressure to perform.
- We become available for joy.
- We soften into gratitude.

Presence is the doorway to contentment. Not because everything is perfect, but because you're finally here for it.

CHOOSE PRESENCE OVER PERFECTION

From Performance to Peace

Perfection says: *"You have to do more to matter."*
Presence says: *"You already matter. Slow down and live."*

As a happiness coach, I've seen clients completely turn their lives around, not by achieving more, but by learning how to be here more.

They start asking different questions:
- *"What does this moment need from me?"*
- *"How do I want to feel, right now?"*
- *"What am I grateful for, even if nothing has changed?"*

And just like that, the frantic becomes sacred. The rush becomes reverence. The mind unclenches, and the heart opens.

Simple Ways to Practice Presence

Here are a few powerful ways to anchor yourself in the now:

1. The 5 Senses Reset

Wherever you are, pause and notice:
- 5 things you can see
- 4 things you can touch
- 3 things you can hear
- 2 things you can smell
- 1 thing you can taste

This is a quick way to return to your body—and the moment.

2. Single-Task with Intention

Instead of multitasking, choose to do one thing slowly.
Drink your tea and *only* drink your tea.
Walk without your phone.
Fold laundry while listening to music—not checking email.
Presence is in the pauses.

CHOOSE PRESENCE OVER PERFECTION

3. Let It Be Imperfect

When something doesn't go as planned, breathe.
Smile.
Say to yourself, *"It's okay. Life isn't perfect, but it's still beautiful."*

A Note on Comparison

Perfectionism often rides on the back of comparison.
You scroll through other people's highlight reels and wonder if your ordinary is enough.

But here's the thing, **your joy is not behind someone else's filter.**
It's not in their career path, their body type, or their curated kitchen. It's in your real, *messy*, beautiful life. Being present allows you to see what's right in front of you, not just what you think you're missing.

A Happiness Coach's Insight
You don't have to earn the right to rest.
You don't need to prove your worth through perfect outcomes.
And you are never behind in a life that's yours alone to live.

Freedom comes when you give yourself permission to be fully human.

And being fully human means being here:
- In the laughter and the tears
- In the joy and the discomfort
- In the now

Because now is all we ever really have.

Perfection will always ask you to perform.
Presence will always invite you to *be*.

When you choose presence over perfection, you
no longer have to chase your life.
You get to live it.

In the next chapter, we'll learn to Follow What
Feels Light, and how your joy can become your
compass out of the cage and into freedom.

REFLECTION EXERCISE: FROM PRESSURE TO PRESENCE

1. What is one area of your life where you feel pressure to be perfect?
Write it down without judgment.

2. How has this pressure affected your peace, your joy, or your relationships?

3. Now ask yourself: What would it feel like to just show up imperfectly—but fully present—in this area?

4. Create a mantra to remind you:
"I release the pressure to be perfect.
 I choose to be here—whole, human, and enough."

Put it somewhere you'll see it every day.

_____

_____

_____

_____

_____

_____

_____

_____

_____

_____

_____

_____

_____

_____

_____

_____

_____

"The subconscious stores. The Observer sees. But together, they help us remember who we are and notice when we've forgotten."

SHANI T. NIGHT

MIDPOINT REFLECTION

THE THREE VERSIONS OF YOU:
A SOULFUL REFRAME OF SELF

MIDPOINT REFLECTION

As we journey through the process of uncaging the mind, it's important to pause and notice the different parts of ourselves that have emerged along the way.

1. The Observer – Awareness
   • This represents the first essential step: Recognize the Cage.
   • The Observer is pure awareness—the version of you that sees without judgment, that witnesses the patterns, fears, and inner dialogues keeping you stuck.
   • This part of you is essential to start the uncaging process. It's the still voice that says, "There's more to me than this."

The Observer is your quiet awareness—the still presence that watches your life unfold without judgment. This is your inner anchor.

2. The Interpreter – Acceptance + Meaning-making
   • This aligns with Challenge the Narrative, Cultivate Self-Compassion, and Choose Presence Over Perfection.
   • The Interpreter is how we give meaning to our stories—how we rewrite inherited beliefs, decode past programming, and choose new truths. Helping you understand that you can reshape your narrative and move from shame to self-compassion.

The Interpreter gives meaning to your experiences—turning moments into beliefs, stories, and lessons. This is the storyteller within.

MIDPOINT REFLECTION

As we journey through the process of uncaging the mind, it's important to pause and notice the different parts of ourselves that have emerged along the way.

3. The Connector – Soulful Living
- This is your final stage: Alignment and Action.
- The Connector is the free, thriving version of self who chooses joy, builds healthy relationships, expands into new spaces, and lives from a place of purpose.
- This part of us seeks light, community, expansion, and presence, everything we will celebrate in the next chapters.

The Connector reaches outward—loving, giving, and finding resonance with others. This is the part of you that seeks soulful living through relationship, purpose, and presence.

These are not masks, but energies. They are movements of your soul. Each plays a role in your uncaging.

MIDPOINT REFLECTION EXERCISE

Before You Begin This Reflection...

This journaling prompt invites you to connect with the deeper layers of your inner self—not to judge or fix, but to simply notice.

The "three versions of self" are not rigid roles or labels. Instead, they are gentle ways to understand how you move through the world:

One part watches (Observer)
One part makes meaning (Interpreter)
One part reaches out and connects (Connector)
Each has wisdom. Each plays a role in your growth.

Example:
Let's say you recently had a difficult conversation.

- The *Observer* in you might have noticed your body tensing up or the urge to stay quiet.
- The *Interpreter* might have thought, "They don't really hear me," drawing on past stories.
- The *Connector* in you may have still shown up with compassion, hoping to bridge the gap.

By reflecting in this way, you'll begin to see how you respond, what old patterns might be showing up, and how you can choose your freedom going forward.

Take your time. Be honest. And most importantly, be kind to yourself.

MIDPOINT REFLECTION EXERCISE

1. When do I feel most like the Observer? What has my quiet awareness taught me lately?
2. What stories am I currently interpreting about my life? Are they helping me grow or keeping me caged?
3. Where and how am I reaching out as the Connector? Who or what am I being called to connect with more deeply?

Let this be a sacred pause. A mirror. A checkpoint between who you've been and who you're becoming.

ALIGNMENT

Alignment is the harmony between who you are, what you believe, and how you live.

From a happiness coach's perspective, **alignment happens when your thoughts, values, actions, and purpose all move in the same direction.** It's when you stop living for expectations and start living from your truth.

Here's what alignment looks and feels like:
- You **say yes** to what fuels your soul and no to what drains it
- Your **values guide your decisions**—not pressure, fear, or people-pleasing
- You feel **peaceful, energized, and clear** about your direction
- You're no longer chasing happiness—**you're embodying it**

✦ *When you're in alignment, life doesn't feel like a constant struggle—it flows.* You're not fighting to be someone else. You're simply being **you**, fully and unapologetically.

Think of it this way:
Alignment is when your **inner world** and your **outer life** are finally speaking the same language.

CHAPTER 5:
FOLLOW WHAT FEELS LIGHT

FOLLOW WHAT FEELS LIGHT

There's a quiet wisdom inside you.
It whispers—not shouts.

It says: *"This feels good."*
"This energizes me."
"This brings me joy."

But for many of us, we've learned to ignore that voice.
We were taught to follow what's **expected**, not what feels **light**.

Yet lightness is not laziness.
It's not irresponsibility.
It's the soul's way of showing you where freedom lives.

The Language of Lightness

Lightness is energy.
You feel it when something:
- Makes you smile without effort
- Sparks curiosity or peace
- Feels like ease—not struggle
- Leaves you feeling *more* alive, not drained

It's the feeling of alignment. But most of us have been conditioned to trust *logic* over *lightness*. We do what makes sense on paper. We follow the "safe" route, the "right" choice, the path of approval. And while those choices might keep us secure... they can also keep us stuck.

FOLLOW WHAT FEELS LIGHT

Heavy Doesn't Always Mean Holy

There's a cultural lie that says:
If it doesn't hurt, it's not worth it.
If it's not hard, it's not valuable.
If it's not a struggle, it's not real.

But not every breakthrough has to come from a breakdown.
Not every blessing requires burnout.

What if ease was a sign of alignment—not weakness?
What if joy was a green light instead of a guilty pleasure?

You don't have to suffer your way to success.
You can follow what lifts you.
You can follow what feels like *freedom*.

Your Inner Compass

As a happiness coach, one of the most powerful shifts I help people make is learning to trust their **inner compass** again.

They begin to notice:
- What drains them
- What inspires them
- What their body says "yes" to
- What makes them breathe easier

The more they pay attention, the clearer their path becomes.

Joy is intelligent.
It's not random.
It's direction.

FOLLOW WHAT FEELS LIGHT

Questions to Find the Light

To begin following what feels light, ask yourself:
- *What gives me energy, even on tired days?*
- *What am I doing when I feel most "me"?*
- *What conversations light me up? What people leave me inspired?*
- *Where do I feel freedom? Ease? Flow?*

Then take one small step toward more of that.

Lightness doesn't mean your life will be free of challenges.
But it **does** mean you'll be fueled by purpose, not pressure.

What Lightness Feels Like

You might feel light when:
- Walking in nature
- Writing, painting, creating
- Laughing deeply with someone who sees you
- Teaching, helping, or serving in a way that aligns with your values
- Dancing in your kitchen, barefoot and free

That feeling? That's your soul stretching its wings.
That's your truth, uncluttered by fear.

You were never meant to feel caged by your own life.

FOLLOW WHAT FEELS LIGHT

But What About Responsibility?

Let's be clear, this isn't about abandoning your obligations or pretending life is always easy.

It's about **balance**.
It's about choosing energy over exhaustion whenever possible.
It's about asking: "*Is there a lighter way to do this?*"

Sometimes the light thing is still hard, like ending a toxic relationship, setting a boundary, or saying no. But even those things can feel like relief... like a deep exhale... like truth. Lightness isn't the absence of effort. It's the presence of *alignment*.

A Happiness Coach's Insight

When you follow what feels light:

- You reconnect with your intuition.
- You find clarity without overthinking.
- You attract opportunities that align with your soul.
- You become magnetic, not because you're perfect, but because you're free.

The heaviness lifts, not all at once, but gradually.
The cage loosens.
And you begin to soar.

"Your journal is not a place for perfection —it's a mirror for your truth and a container for your freedom."

SHANI T. NIGHT

REFLECTION EXERCISE: WHAT FEELS LIGHT?

1. Make a Light vs. Heavy List.

Draw a line down the middle of a page.

Label one side "Light" and the other "Heavy."

On the *Light* side, list the things, people, places, and habits that make you feel energized, joyful, and alive.

On the *Heavy* side, list what feels draining, forced, or misaligned.

Light	Heavy

"You don't have to earn your freedom
—you just have to remember it's
already yours."

Shani T. Night

REFLECTION EXERCISE: WHAT FEELS LIGHT?

2. Ask: What can I do less of from the heavy side?
What can I invite more of from the light?

3. Choose one "light" action this week.
Call the friend who lifts your spirit.
Take the walk.
Say no to the draining obligation.
Do the thing that feels like sunshine in your chest.

Joy is not a luxury.
It's your **birthright.**
Lightness is not a detour.
It's your **true direction.**

You don't need permission to feel good.
You need permission to trust *yourself* again.

And in the next chapter, we'll explore what happens when you **Surround Yourself with Expansion**—because you were never meant to grow in a cage.

CHAPTER 6:
SURROUND YOURSELF WITH EXPANSION

SURROUND YOURSELF WITH EXPANSION

When you're in a cage long enough, the walls start to feel like home. They trick you into thinking that what's small is safe. That shrinking is security. But deep down, you were made to grow.

To uncage your mind, you must surround yourself with *expansion*—people, places, and perspectives that stretch you, inspire you, and remind you how vast your life can be.

You Become What You're Around

We're like emotional sponges. Without realizing it, we absorb the energy, mindset, and language of our environment.

If you're around people who complain constantly, you'll start to echo their frustrations.
If you're surrounded by fear, you'll play it safe.
If you're exposed only to the past, you'll forget to dream forward.

But the opposite is also true:
If you spend time with dreamers, healers, doers, and thinkers...

You'll start to rise.

SURROUND YOURSELF WITH EXPANSION

Expansion Feels Like Possibility

Expansion isn't about being busier. It's about being **bigger** inside. It's that moment when someone says something that clicks deep in your soul. Or when you're in a space that makes you whisper, "*I didn't know it could feel this good.*"

You might find expansion in:
- A book that challenges your beliefs
- A friend who sees greatness in you
- A mentor who's walked the path you dream of
- A new place that wakes something up inside you
- A community that encourages growth over perfection

Expansion is nourishment for your soul.

The Power of Conversations

Some conversations shrink you.
They keep you tethered to gossip, complaints, and fear.
They keep you rehearsing your pain instead of releasing it.

Other conversations *grow* you.
They spark ideas. They offer hope. They make you feel brave.
They don't focus on who you were, but on *who you're becoming*.

Ask yourself:
- Who do I talk to that makes me feel *seen* and *safe*?
- Who challenges me in healthy, loving ways?
- Who helps me think bigger, feel better, and dream wider?

These are your *expansion allies*—your tribe of light.

SURROUND YOURSELF WITH EXPANSION

Change Your Room, Change Your View

Sometimes, to think differently, you need to **stand somewhere new.**

Nature expands you.
So does art, music, and movement.
Travel expands you—so does silence.
A well-timed podcast or even a simple walk through a bookstore can crack your heart wide open.

You don't always need a plane ticket. Sometimes all it takes is walking into a space where your *soul feels taller.*

Outgrowing Isn't Disloyalty

This part is hard. Because sometimes the people, spaces, or conversations you outgrow are the ones you love the most.

But let me be gentle and honest:

Growth will make you uncomfortable before it makes you unstoppable.

You are not betraying your past by moving forward.
You're honoring your future.

You're not better than the people you're outgrowing, you're just *becoming different.*

And different doesn't have to mean distant.
It just means intentional.

SURROUND YOURSELF WITH EXPANSION

Curate Your Circle

Here's your permission slip:

You are allowed to choose who and what gets access to your mind, time, and energy.

Ask yourself:
- Does this connection breathe life into me?
- Do I feel more *me* around them—or less?
- Are we growing in the same direction?

You deserve to be in rooms where:
- Growth is celebrated, not judged
- Vulnerability is strength, not shame
- Joy is contagious, not questioned

Protect your peace. Prioritize your potential.

A Coach's Truth: You Grow at the Edges

When I work with clients, their biggest breakthroughs don't come from doing more. They come from being **more intentional** with their surroundings.

I've watched people change their lives just by:
- Saying yes to one retreat
- Joining one uplifting group
- Reading one life-changing book
- Letting go of one toxic relationship

Growth doesn't always require a revolution—sometimes it just takes *rearranging the furniture of your life* to face the window, not the wall.

ACTION

Action is the bridge between intention and transformation.

From a happiness coach's perspective, **action** is how we turn our dreams, values, and inner work into real, visible change in our lives. It's not just about doing, it's about doing with purpose.

Action is:
- **The courage to move** even when the path isn't clear
- **The follow-through** on what you say matters to you
- **The daily choices** that align with your joy, healing, and growth
- **Energy in motion -**your beliefs, values, and goals expressed through behavior

You can *read* about growth. You can *talk* about change. You can *hope* for a better life.

But it's **action** that takes you there.
It's the **yes** you say to yourself.
It's the **step** you take, even if it's small.

✨*Clarity comes through action.* Confidence is built in the doing. If happiness is a garden, then action is how you plant, water, and grow it.

REFLECTION EXERCISE: WHO AND WHAT EXPANDS YOU?

1. Name 3 people in your life who help you feel limitless, alive, and seen.

2. Name 3 spaces—physical or virtual—where you feel inspired and at peace.

3. Name 3 things you can expose yourself to this month (a class, a conversation, a book, a new place) that challenge you to grow.

Then commit to *one step* this week.
Let the light in.
Let the small cage crack open.

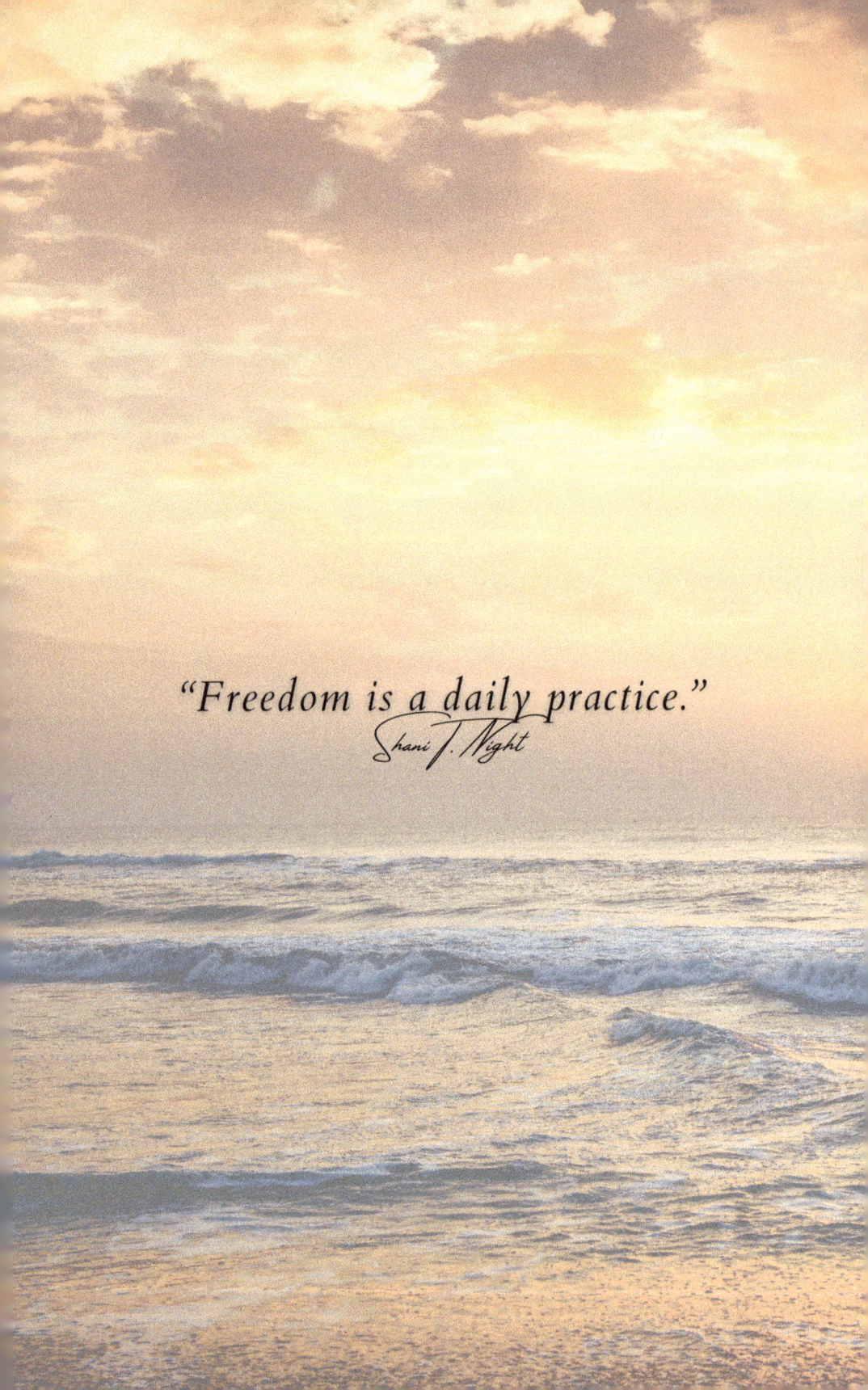

"Freedom is a daily practice."

Shani T. Night

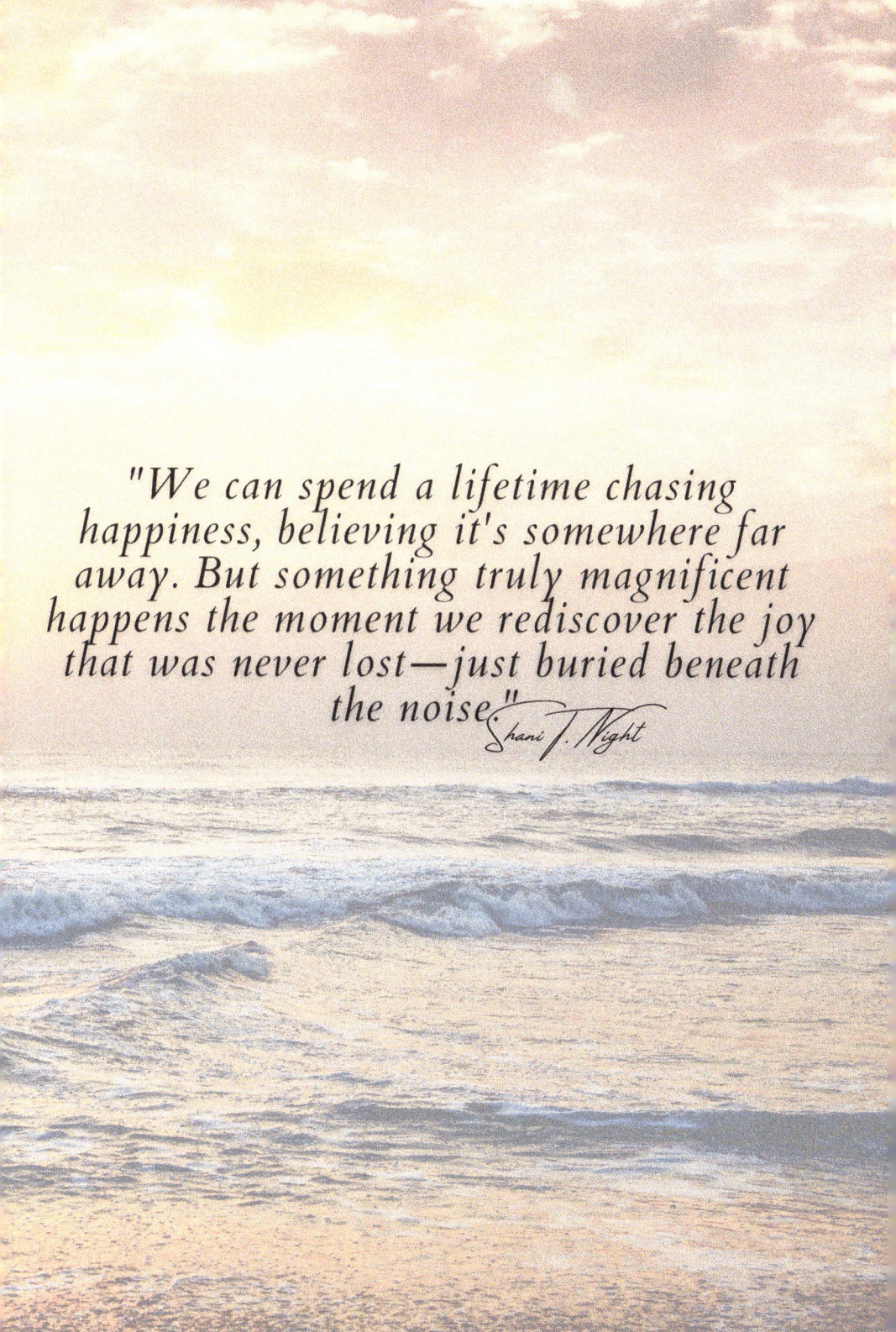

"We can spend a lifetime chasing happiness, believing it's somewhere far away. But something truly magnificent happens the moment we rediscover the joy that was never lost—just buried beneath the noise." *Shani T. Night*

You are not meant to live small.
You are not meant to repeat old cycles.
You are not meant to feel stuck.

You were made for *expansion*.
And the more you surround yourself with what lifts you, the more naturally you rise.

In the next chapter, we'll explore what it really means to practice freedom daily, because uncaging your mind isn't a one-time moment... it's a way of life.

CHAPTER 7:
FREEDOM IS A DAILY PRACTICE

FREEDOM IS A DAILY PRACTICE

Freedom is not a finish line. It's not a mountaintop you reach and then descend, changed forever. It's a choice. A rhythm. A return.

You don't uncage your mind once and then you're done. You uncage it **again and again**—each time fear whispers, each time doubt rises, each time the old you tries to pull you back.

The truth is, *freedom is a daily practice.*

You Wake Up With Keys in Your Pocket

Every morning, you are handed a choice:

Will I stay in the cage of comfort and limitation today?
Or will I use my keys—awareness, compassion, presence, joy, truth—to unlock something greater?

Some days, freedom looks like speaking up.
Other days, it looks like resting when the world says grind.
Some days, it means choosing forgiveness.
Other days, it's walking away.

Freedom doesn't always roar.
Sometimes it whispers, *"Not today, fear. I'm choosing me."*

FREEDOM IS A DAILY PRACTICE

Old Thoughts Visit—Don't Move Back In

Here's what most people don't realize:

Freedom isn't the absence of limiting thoughts.
It's the ability to *notice them and not believe them anymore.*

That voice in your head might say:
- "You're not doing enough."
- "What if you mess this up?"
- "Who do you think you are?"

And your response is not to fight it, but to smile gently and say:
"Thank you for your opinion, but I'm choosing differently today."

Every time you meet that voice with love instead of panic, you strengthen your freedom muscle.

Small Choices = Big Liberation

You don't need grand gestures to be free.

Freedom is in the *micro-moments*:

- Taking a breath before reacting.
- Saying no to something that drains you.
- Drinking water instead of numbing out.
- Journaling your truth instead of bottling it.
- Walking in nature instead of scrolling.

These are small decisions. But they say, I *matter. I choose presence. I choose peace.* They add up.

FREEDOM IS A DAILY PRACTICE

Create a Daily Freedom Ritual

As a happiness coach, I always remind my clients: **what you do daily, you become.** If you want to become free, create *rituals* that anchor you in freedom.

Here are a few powerful ones:

Morning Intention: Start your day with an affirmation.
- "Today, I choose truth over fear."
- "Today, I show up fully as myself."

Midday Reset: Set a reminder to pause and check-in.
- Where am I feeling caged? What would feel freeing right now?

Evening Reflection: Ask yourself:
- "What did freedom look like for me today?"
- "Where did I show up courageously?"
- "What can I let go of before tomorrow?"

Your day doesn't need perfection—it needs *presence*.

FREEDOM IS A DAILY PRACTICE

Repetition Is Power, Not Failure

If you find yourself battling the same limiting beliefs, don't get discouraged. That's not failure, it's part of the practice.

Think of freedom like brushing your teeth. You don't do it once and never again, you return to it, over and over, because *you're worth it.*

So when the fear comes back, or the inner critic gets loud again, don't panic.

Just return to what you know:

- You are not your thoughts.
- You are not your past.
- You are not your fear.
- You are free, even when you forget.

Forgive Yourself—Daily

Real freedom includes the ability to forgive yourself quickly.

If you snap, overthink, fall into comparison, or shrink back—don't linger there.

A caged mind punishes itself.
A free mind says, *"That wasn't my highest self, but I'm learning. I still love me."*

Each time you offer yourself grace, you unlock another door.

"When realization and actualization meet, you awaken to the knowing of who you are—worthy, whole, and finally able to appreciate the beauty of your becoming."

SHANI T. NIGHT

FREEDOM IS A DAILY PRACTICE

Stay Close to Your Tools

Freedom is fragile when we forget our tools.

Keep them nearby:

- Your affirmations
- Your gratitude practice
- Your breath
- Your boundaries
- Your support system
- Your dreams

Think of these as your keys. When things feel heavy or tight, reach for them. Use them.

Because your freedom is not only possible—it's *your natural state.*

"I may not have lived many lifetimes, but I've lived many versions of myself—and each chapter, in its beauty and its breaking, has led me brilliantly to this moment of truth and purpose."

SHANI T. NIGHT

"I may not have lived many lives, but I've poured my heart into living one life brilliantly."

SHANI T. NIGHT

"The most powerful person is the one who knows their worth and owns it."

SHANI T. NIGHT

Freedom isn't loud or flashy.
It's not perfection or constant joy.
It's not the absence of fear.

Freedom is waking up and deciding—one mindful, beautiful moment at a time—that you're no longer available for smallness, shame, or settling.

It's choosing your truth again and again, even when it shakes your voice.
It's choosing your joy, even when it's inconvenient.
It's choosing your worth, even when the world tells you otherwise.

Freedom is a daily practice.

And the more you practice, the more natural it becomes.

Daily Freedom Journal Prompt:

What would freedom look like for me *today*?
What one choice can I make right now that honors my truth?

You don't have to change everything all at once.
Just take one free step.
Then another.
And another.

Until you look around one day and realize:
You are no longer in the cage.
You are home—inside yourself.

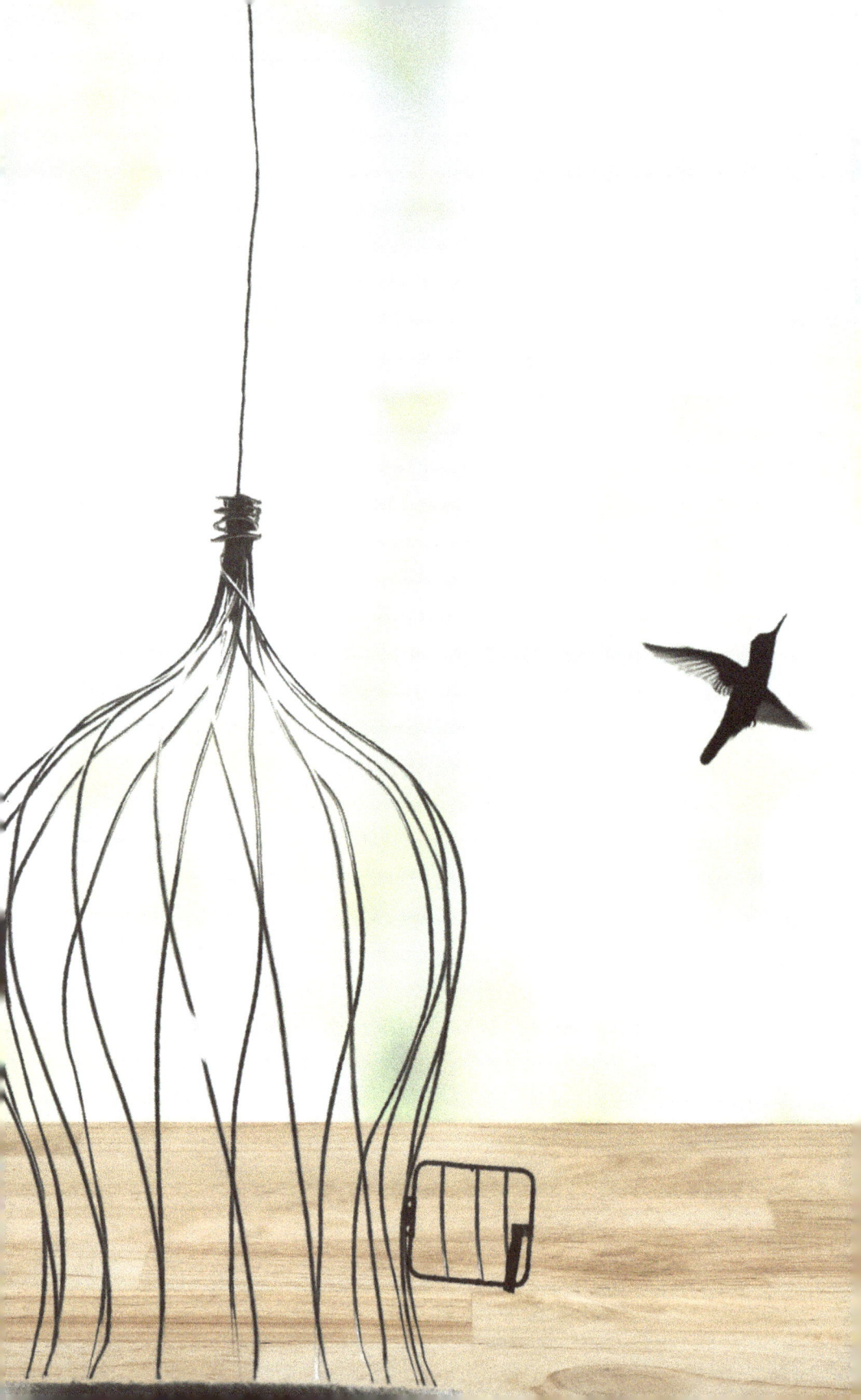

A COACH'S CLOSING WORD

Dear Reader,

If you've made it to this point, I want to honor the brave and beautiful work you've done—reading, reflecting, opening, and unlearning. That alone is a form of freedom.

This book was never about fixing you—because you were never broken. It was about remembering the truth of who you are beneath the noise, the masks, the fear, and the expectations. It was about helping you find the courage to live with intention, peace, and purpose. To uncage the mind and come home to the soul.

You've been surviving for a long time. Now it's time to live.
Not on autopilot. Not by someone else's script. But with joy, clarity, and authenticity. Freedom isn't a finish line, it's a practice. And now you have the tools, the awareness, and the heart to keep choosing it, every single day.

Let this be your reminder:
You are allowed to change.
You are allowed to grow.
You are allowed to be joyful.
You are allowed to be free.

I'm proud of you.
I'm rooting for you.
And I'll meet you in every moment where truth and joy intersect.

With love and light,
Shani T. Night
Your Happiness Coach and Fellow Traveler

About the Author

My mission as a certified Happiness Life Wellness Coach is to help individuals live their happiest, healthiest, and most fulfilling lives. I believe that true happiness comes from within, and that by making positive changes in our thoughts, behaviors, and lifestyle, we can transform our lives and achieve lasting well-being.

I am committed to providing personalized coaching that is tailored to the unique needs and goals of each individual client. I believe that everyone has the potential to be happy and successful, and that my role is to provide guidance, support, and encouragement as my clients work to achieve their dreams.

I believe that wellness is a holistic concept that encompasses physical, emotional, and spiritual health, and that by addressing all aspects of wellness, we can achieve a more balanced and fulfilling life. Through my coaching, I aim to empower my clients to take control of their well-being and to make positive changes that will last a lifetime.

My goal is to create a safe, supportive, and non-judgmental space where my clients can explore their thoughts and feelings, overcome their challenges, and discover their true potential. I am passionate about helping others live their best lives, and I am dedicated to making a positive difference in the world, one client at a time.

From the Author

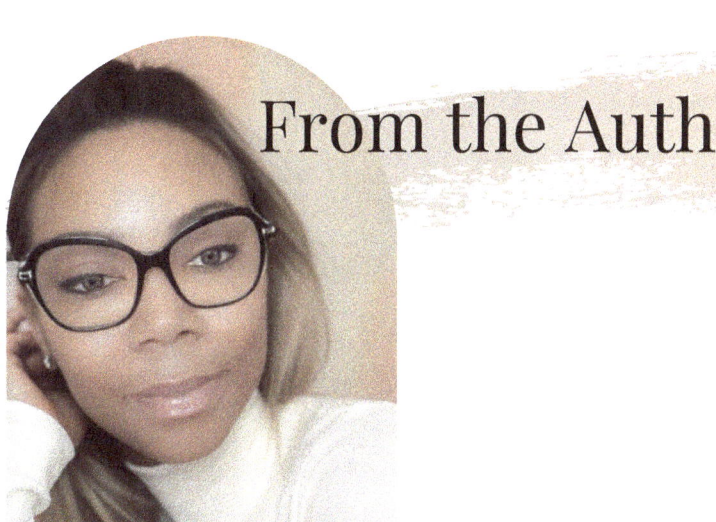

For me, happiness is finding contentment in my own skin, regardless of my location. It's embracing the radiance I emit and the positive energy I embody. True happiness lies in simply existing, free from the constraints of comparison or competition. It's about embracing both the favorable and challenging aspects of life and consistently embodying grace, compassion, and love. It involves acknowledging the inherent goodness in people, embracing them without judgment, and trusting a higher power to handle judgment while striving to be the best version of myself.

Moreover, it's recognizing that as a reflection of light, truth, compassion, grace, and love, I have the potential to positively impact those around me. I may serve as a beacon of inspiration, guiding others toward a better path and offering a source of light and support to those who need it. This awareness adds depth to my happiness, knowing that my journey is not only about personal fulfillment but also about contributing positively to the well-being of others.

Books by Shani

Introspective books guide us through the complexity of our thoughts, emotions, and behaviors. They ask the hard questions—**Why do I react this way? What do I truly value? What's driving my choices?**—and help us explore the answers.

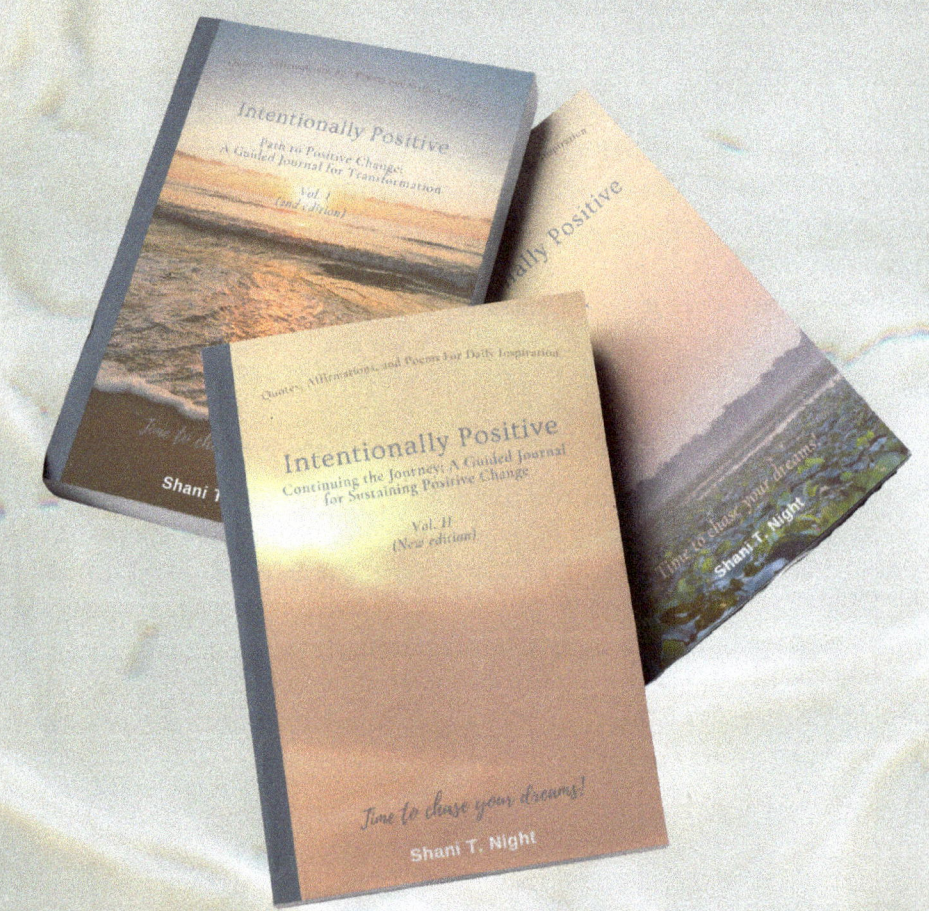

When we write, we pause. We process. We purge. Whether it's pain, confusion, dreams, or breakthroughs, journaling gives them a home. Over time, it becomes a safe space for healing and clarity.

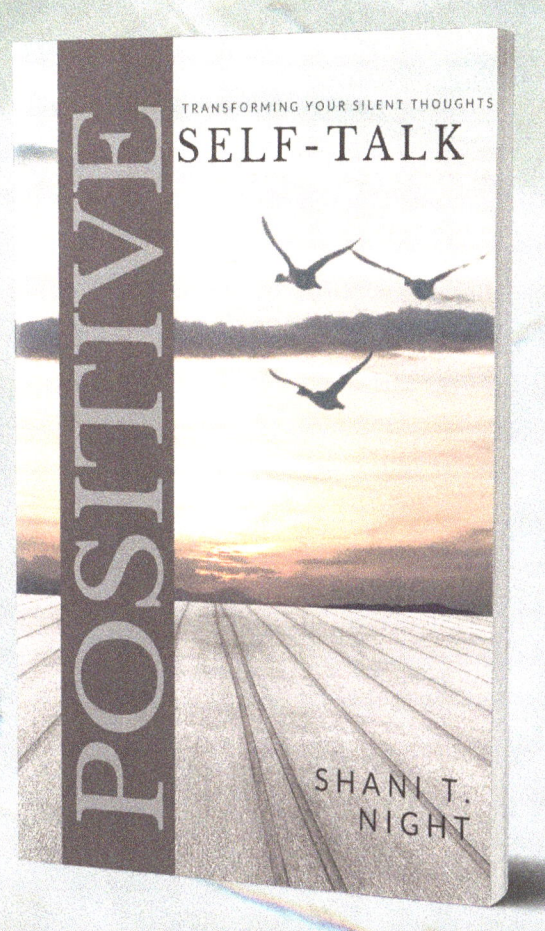

"The key to happiness first starts with you and you alone."

SHANI T. NIGHT

Knowing who you are is
it's own
appreciation.
SHANI T. NIGHT

www.ingramcontent.com/pod-product-compliance
Lightning Source LLC
Chambersburg PA
CBHW051328120626
46547CB00015B/2444

* 9 7 8 1 9 5 3 3 6 4 7 4 6 *